I0416369

More Taste Less Waist!

By

Chad Shaw

ISBN: 978-1-312-72611-6

© Chad Shaw 2014, all rights reserved.

Photography © Desirée Duggan, Corso Photographic 2014. All rights reserved.
www.ChadShaw.net
www.CorsoPhoto.com

Table of Contents

Chapter 5: Drinks and Shakes

Chapter 6: Pizzas

Chapter 7: Breads and Desserts

Foreword

The subject of nutrition is the most viciously debated topic in the world of fitness. As confusing as the subject of nutrition is for so many people; the premise of nutrition is actually quite simple. It took me many years to figure this out myself. When various bodybuilding and fitness periodicals published articles regarding the best type of nutrition to support muscle building and fat loss, they always seem to promote these bland, boring diets involving these very militant eating regimens that consisted of the exact same boring foods being consumed over and over again, every single day. They seemed to reflect the idea that food was strictly a means to an end, but not something should be enjoyed. The whole ideology that suggests "if it tastes good, then spit it out because it will make you fat!"

I've got news for everyone: Your body does not decide what foods that it will or will not store as fat based on how good the food tastes! Your body stores or burns fat based on the amount of energy that you feed it. When you consume calories that exceed your body's energy and metabolic requirements on any given day, then your body will store those excess calories as fat. Anytime that you feed your body fewer calories than it requires in order to fulfill its energy and metabolic requirements, then your body has no choice but to begin burning stored body fat in order to compensate for that energy deficit that was created by the decrease in calorie consumption.

Additionally, I've been experimenting with various diets for several decades and discovered that you can create some extremely savory meals that will not only satisfy particular food cravings, but also help you adhere to a reduced calorie diet that will lead to the loss of body fat. Of course the key is to understand serving sizes so that you don't accidentally consume too many calories and derail your weight loss efforts. This is why I made the decision to take the guess work out of this for you by breaking down the serving sizes of each recipe for you and provide the nutritional information for each of them as well. This will allow you to strategically incorporate some of these great tasting foods into your diet so that you don't feel deprived, yet still be able to effectively obtain your fitness goals.

The number one reason why most people fail on diets is because most fat loss diets involve some type of extreme deprivation. When people attempt to adhere to these types of diets, they inevitably begin to feel deprived and run-down. Not to mention, they feel like they're missing out when they look around witness everyone else around them eating all this delicious tasting food. Eventually all of these feelings come to a head and these people abandon their diets all together and make a fast transition into binge eating; in an attempt to make up for weeks or months of nutritional deprivation. Of course, we all know where binge eating gets us. Right back to square one! It's a vicious cycle that is tough to break. However, I believe that the recipes contained in this book will help people break the vicious cycle, so that they can reach their fitness goals without feeling like they're missing out on the joy that is associated with eating great tasting food!   ~Chad Shaw

All throughout my childhood, I have always felt slightly on the chubby side. Not fat, but certainly not athletic. After graduating High school and moving out of my house, I decided to make it a point to learn how to eat and how to lose weight. I ended up losing more weight than I had ever imagined and going from 5'6" and 148 pounds 112 pounds. I hovered around that weight until deciding to put on muscle to look like the girls in the fitness magazines and now I feel healthier and stronger than ever. I have accrued a lifetime of tweaking existing recipes with healthier ingredients, including some old family favorites like my mother's sauce. After moving in with Chad in October of 2013 and realizing he did the exact same thing that I did with tweaking recipes, we decided that we really needed to share this information with the world!
As a fitness photographer, I decided to start photographing each meal as it came out of the oven or off the stove, and over the course of nine months this book came together as if by magic. We began posting a recipe here and there on Chad's website or in his monthly newsletter, and realized we had enough recipes to create an actual cookbook. I have been so privileged to enjoy participating in food photography as photo shoots take only five to ten minutes to compete and you can eat the subjects!
Just knowing this book has the information to help people change their lives for the better made it a joy to create. Bon Appatit my friends!
~ Desirée Duggan

Recipes are given one, two, or three asterisks (*) on the title as to how easy they are to prepare. One asterisk (*) = very quick and easy, two asterisks (**) = typical meal cooking time, or three (***) which means there may be a short prep time but long cooking time, or may be a bit more involved to make; and finally four (****) for those who love to cook. However, the three and four star dishes tend to be larger and will feed you over a longer period of time as leftovers, which are the easiest dinners of all!

Chapter 1: Breakfast Foods

High Protein Pancakes **
1/4 cup of almond flour
1/4 cup of flax meal
1 scoop of vanilla whey protein
3 whole eggs
1/4 cup of plain Greek yogurt
1/3 cup of almond milk
1/4 cup of chopped fresh fruit of your choice (optional, add calories).
1/4 cup of whole wheat flour
*for gluten free pancakes substitute the wheat flour with quinoa flour

 Mix all ingredients together in a medium sized bowl. Mix dry ingredients first, followed by the wet ingredients, then add wet ingredients to the dry and combine them together to form pancake batter. Mix thoroughly until smooth. Heat pan to a medium heat and spray pan with non-fat cooking spray. This recipe makes approximately 8, 5-inch pancakes.
Each pancake: 90 calories,   8 g protein   4 g fat   4 g carb   1.5 g fiber

Pumpkin pancakes**

1/2 cup of almond flour
2 TBSP of ground flax seed
1 serving of vanilla whey protein
1/3 cup of canned pumpkin
1 cage free egg
4 egg whites
1/4 cup of unsweetened almond milk
1 tsp of cinnamon
1 tsp of all spice
1/2 tsp of ginger
1 tsp of vanilla extract

In a medium sized bowl, add and thoroughly mix the ingredients.
Preheat skillet, or frying pan to a medium heat. Coat skillet, or pan with non-fat cooking spray.
Using a large spoon, scoop a portion of the pancake batter onto skillet, or frying pan to form the pancakes. Use the spoon to form pancake into the desired shape. Let cook for approximately 5 minutes, or until large

pores begin to form on the upright side of the pancakes. Using a spatula, flip the pancakes over to cook the opposite sides. Let them cook for approximately 3 minutes, or until the pancakes are cooked all the way through. Divide pancakes and top with sugar free syrup, or favorite low calorie topping. To avoid aspartame, we suggest using Smucker's sugar free breakfast syrup or Walden Farms sugar free syrup.

Makes 8 pancakes   (Each)   86 calories   5g fat   7.5g protein   3g carb   1.5g fiber

French Toast *

2 slices Ezekiel or Julian Bread (Julian Bread has 1g net carb)
½ cup better than eggs or egg whites
Sugar free Maple syrup if desired
1 tsp Cinnamon
Sweetener of choice (if desired. Not sugar, equal, or saccharin)
1 tsp vanilla extract
Nonstick cooking spray

Pour egg substitute in a shallow bowl or high sided plate. Add 1 tsp vanilla extract, 1 packet sweetener (we prefer the green-stevia, or the orange-monk fruit), and ½ tsp cinnamon, whip with fork. Spray pan with nonstick cooking spray, put pan to warm for 1 minute on medium heat. Dredge bread slices in egg mixture then put in pan. Cook until golden brown on each side, then put on plate, add a small amount of sugar free syrup and the other ½ tsp cinnamon.

Total:
Julian Paleo almond Bread   213 calories   20 g protein   6g fat
13g carb   5g fiber
Ezekiel Bread   253 calories   17g protein   1.5g fat
26g carb   3g fiber

Protein Chocolate Pudding *

2 scoops Isagenix IsaLean Shake powder: 240 calories 24g protein   6g fat   24g carb   8g fiber
1 package Truvia sweetener
3 tbsps. filtered water
2 tbsp. Monk fruit sweetener or 2 packets Sweetener to taste.
3 tbsps. filtered water

In a bowl, add shake powder, then add 1 tbsp. water and whip with a spoon for 30 seconds. If this does not allow all of the powder to assimilate, then add another tablespoon of water and whip with spoon. Keep whipping and adding small amounts of water until it reaches desired consistency. When adding sweeteners, add one by one and stir well each time you add it and take a small taste so you can make it as sweet as you want it, then remember what you used so you can add the sweetener to the dry ingredients next time.

For a variation, add some PB2 peanut butter powder for that peanut butter cup taste! It will add a few extra calories.

While pudding is not typically classified as a breakfast food, we chose to put it here because it is a nutritionally complete meal and will keep you full and satisfied. When eaten with an 8 ounce glass of water, it will be too heavy for eating after dinner as a dessert.

Tropical Toast with Protein Pina Colada *

2 slices Ezekiel or Julian Bread
1 tbsp. extra virgin coconut oil
1/8 cup unsweetened coconut shavings
1 scoop vanilla protein
½ cup water
4-5 medium ice cubes
½-1 cap full Coconut baking extract
1 tsp vanilla extract
½-1 cap full pineapple baking extract

Toast the two slices of bread in a toaster or toaster oven until light to medium toast, spread on the coconut oil, then sprinkle on the coconut shavings. *to save calories leave out the coconut shavings and use ¼ tsp coconut baking extract and mix it into the coconut oil for flavor.

Coconut Shavings: 55 calories   1g protein   5g fat   4g carb
Coconut Oil: 130 calories   14g fat
Ezekiel Bread (2 slices): 160 calories   9.6g protein   1g fat   30g carbs   6g fiber

Julian Bakery Paleo Bread (2) 120 calories   14g protein   6g
fat   12g carbs   10g fiber

Total (Ezekiel Bread) 345 calories   10.6g protein   20g fat
34g carbs

Total (Julian Bread)   305 calories   15g protein   25g fat
16g carbs (5g net carbs)

*Protein Shake: Please view the nutrition information on the
canister of your preferred protein, than add those calories to this
meal. Most proteins are 100-115 calories and 21g protein.

Southwestern Style Veggie Omelet** (Pictured)

Pre-heat a medium to large sized frying pan at a low heat, then
spray pan with non-fat cooking spray.

Place 1-2 cage free eggs in a small bowl with 4 egg whites and
beat eggs until they are blended thoroughly.

Pour eggs into frying pan and allow to cook for a couple of
minutes until eggs begin to solidify.

Place chopped 4 chopped mushrooms, 1/2 cup of chopped
spinach, 1/3 of a medium onion, chopped up, and 1/4 of a green
pepper chopped up, down the center of the cooking eggs. The
veggies should be placed in a long, narrow strip, going down the
center of the eggs.

Sprinkle 1/8 cup of shredded, low-fat cheese on top of the
veggies.

Sprinkle 1/2 tsp of south-western style seasoning, along with 1/4
tsp of black pepper on top of the veggies and cheese.

When eggs appear to be solidified, using a spatula, fold 1 side of
the egg over the top of the veggies and cheese.

Then fold the other side of the egg over the remaining uncovered portion of the veggies and cheese.
Omelet is complete.
To make the omelet more visually appealing, you may sprinkle an additional 1/8 cup of cheese on top of the omelet and place in the oven on a plate at the lowest heat setting, until the cheese is melted on top of the omelet.

Total Calories: 227.5 calories   7.5g fat   30g protein
10.5g carbs   2g fiber

Pair this omelet with a clean carb such as our bagged and baked sweet potato fries, a serving of oatmeal, or a slice or two of Ezekiel bread to start your day.

Chapter 2: Salads & Side Dishes

Peanut Butter Wasabi Salad Dressing *

2 tbsps. Water
2 tbsps. Extra virgin olive oil
1 tsp balsamic vinegar
½ tsp balsamic glaze
½-1 tsp wasabi (not wasabi powder)
2-3 tbsps. PB2 Peanut butter powder

Whip ingredients with a fork in a small bowl. Add peanut butter powder for thickness.
Nice dipping sauce for raw broccoli florets.

Put in refrigerator to thicken if desired. This can be used as a dipping sauce for broccoli and other green vegetables, or an actual salad dressing. If used as a dipping sauce, refrigeration will make it less runny. A thinner dressing is better for a salad so it permeates the entire salad rather than just sitting on the top layer.

Total Calories   256 calories   17.5g
fat   10g protein   19g carb   4g fiber
1 serving (1/4 of the mixture)   64 calories   4.3g
fat   2.5g protein   5g carb   1g fiber

Italian grilled chicken salad **

16 oz. pre-cooked chicken breast, cubed
3 cups cooked whole wheat pasta, rotini or elbows
1 cup zucchini
1 cup broccoli florets diced small
1 can of small artichokes or artichoke quarters
6oz sliced black olives
Fresh basil ½-1 cup
½ onion diced
1 tbsp. oregano
2 cloves garlic pressed or minced from a jar
¼ cup extra virgin olive oil
¼ cup parmesan cheese

Add any other veggies, such as green beans, peppers, cucumber, celery, or spinach as desired.

Total: 8   1841 calories
129g protein   84.4g fat   150.6g carb
Per Serving: 8   230 calories
16g protein   10.6g fat   19g carb

*to add more protein, add a few ounces more of cooked chicken. To reduce fat or calories, use less or no parmesan cheese.

Taco Salad ** (Pictured)

1 lb. ground or cubed chicken, ground turkey, or lean ground beef
1 head of Lettuce
1 can diced tomatoes with chilies
½ pack of reduced fat Mexican cheese
1 avocado
½ onion, diced
1-2 tbsps. Taco seasoning
1 tbsp. chili powder
Black olives and jalapenos if desired
1 tbsp. extra virgin olive oil
1 tsp. balsamic vinegar

Brown ground meat in a skillet sprayed with nonstick spray and mix with taco seasoning, chili powder, and onion.

Simmer on medium-low for 3-5 minutes; add a teaspoon of water if mixture is too dry. When cooking is done, drain water.

Prepare lettuce and toss in the vinegar and oil in a large bowl. Transfer to serving bowls and top with a tablespoon or two of tomatoes with chilies, cheese, ½ avocado, the amount of meat allotted for your diet (typically 4-7 oz.) and black olives.
You can serve with 1 cup of brown rice either mixed in or on the side.

Recipe makes two salads with left overs. Calories are calculated with ground turkey.

Makes 4 servings.

4 oz. ground turkey
¼ avocado
¼ cup tomatoes with chilies
1/8 pack of reduced fat Mexican cheese
1/8 onion
¼ head lettuce
Calories for salad alone: 291 calories   26g protein   19g fat
13g carb   13.4g fiber

Yellow Squash or Zucchini Stir Fry* (Pictured)

1 large zucchini or 2-3 small yellow squash
1 tbsp. grape seed oil
Nonstick cooking spray or grape seed oil cooking spray
Himalayan pink salt or sea salt

Slice squash into ½-3/4" rounds. Spray pan with nonstick cooking spray and pour in ½ tbsp. of the grape seed oil. Let pan heat on medium for a minute or two and hold up pan at an angle so oil spreads around.

Put in squash rounds and cook until they are toasted   and golden brown. Flip them and do the same on the other side. Remove finished squash and add the other ½ tbsp. of grape seed oil and the other rounds that did not fit into the pan.

Serve lightly sprinkled with sea salt if desired.
add 40 cal and 2g fat for oil
Squash/zucchini 20 cal/cup

Bagged and Baked Sweet Potato Fries ** (Pictured)

Take 1-4 sweet potatoes, chop them into either circles, ½ circles, or ¼ circles; put them in a large Ziploc bag with a tablespoon of grape seed or extra virgin olive oil (preferably grape seed because we will be cooking at temps over 350 degrees) add 2 tbsps. of Weber BBQ seasoning, 1 tsp of liquid smoke, ½ tsp of sesame oil, a sprinkle of sea salt, ¼-1/2 tsp garlic powder, and a ¼ tsp black pepper. Shake it and knead it until the spices have made an even coating on the potatoes, spread them out on a foil coated non-stick sprayed cookie sheet and oven bake for 35-40 min @ 400.

Sweet potato: 1 cup   180 calories
4g Protein 0g Fat 41g carb 7g fiber
add 40 cal and 2g fat for oils   220 calories
4g protein 2g fat 41g carb 7g fiber

Have with grilled meat for dinner or with eggs in the morning!

Artichoke Salad **

2 cans artichokes or artichoke hearts
1 can beets
1 8-12 oz. can mushrooms
2 cups cooked whole wheat pasta
2 chopped cucumbers
2 tbsps. Extra virgin olive oil
½ medium red onion
½ cup radish slices
4 scallions
1 can of colossal black olives (12 olives)
½-1 cup fresh chopped basil
2 tbsps. oregano
1 tsp rosemary
½ tsp sea salt
½ tsp black pepper

Total nutrition (whole salad)   943 calories   35g fat
24.9g protein   133.5g carbs   19g fiber

Makes 5 servings; Nutrition for each serving: 189 calories   7g fat
5g protein   27g carbs   4g fiber

Mix dry spices with the olive oil and let sit while you are prepping the rest of the salad. Chop everything and toss in the bowl with the olive oil. For fewer carbs, leave out or reduce the pasta. Serve on the side with a lean meat for lunch or dinner. I call this my "gallbladder salad" because it contains vegetables that support gallbladder function. If you aren't crazy about beets, just know they kind of get lost in the other flavors of the salad. If there is an ingredient you dislike, feel free to remove it and subtract the calories.

Chapter 3: Meats

Upside Down Apple Turkey ***

Turkey is a wonderfully lean meat, and if you put in the cooking time here, this will satisfy you for quite a long time to come. Leftovers can be frozen for convenient meals down the road.

Begin by removing the contents from inside of the turkey, then rinsing off the turkey thoroughly. Peel 3-4 apples
depending on the size of the turkey. For a medium sized turkey use 3 apples, and for a large turkey 4 apples should be enough. The best apples to use are Granny Smith, Pink Lady, or Honey-crisp apples. Cut the peeled apples into slices.

Sprinkle apples slices with cinnamon, and then stuff the apples slices inside of the turkey. Use kitchen string to sew the opening to the turkey body shut so that the apples can't roll out of the turkey.
Rub enough olive oil over the outside of the turkey, so that the entire exterior of the turkey has a light coating of oil on it.

Add your favorite seasonings to the outside of the turkey. Mesquite seasoning with pepper is a great combination, but you can use any seasoning, or turkey rub that you wish to.

Take an oven bag, and follow the baking instructions listed in the oven bag directions. The instructions that come with the over bags will tell you how what temperature to bake the turkey at, and for how long you should bake it, based on the weight of the turkey. A large turkey generally takes close to 3 hours to bake.

Place the turkey in the oven bag and seal the bag with bag tie. Place the turkey breast-side down on a baking pan, and then place in oven to cook for the required amount of time.

When turkey has finished baking, remove turkey from oven, and let turkey cool for about 15 minutes.
Lastly, open up the oven bag and use a spoon to removed baked apple slices from the turkey. Slice up the turkey, and serve with apple slices on the turkey.

Turkey Breast: 5 ounces 150 calories   2g fat   22g protein
3g carbs
Turkey Dark Meat: 4 ounces   212 calories   8g fat   32g
protein   ---carbs

Grilled BBQ Chicken Breast

Preheat grill to about 400 degrees.
Take 16 oz. of chicken breasts (approximately 4 chicken breasts) and place them in a 1 gallon sized plastic food storage bag.

In the food storage bag, along with the chicken; add: 1 tbsp. of extra virgin olive oil, 2 tsp of liquid smoke, 1 tbsp. of McCormick Grill Mate Barbecue seasoning, 1 tsp of Black pepper, and 1 tsp of Mesquite seasoning.

Next, seal the food storage bag and shake up with all of the contents inside. Work your hands around the outside of the bag, to roll the chicken breast in the bag, so that all of the pieces of chicken are evenly coated by the seasonings and oil inside of the bag.

Remove the pieces of chicken from the bag, and strategically place each piece of chicken on the grill so that each piece will cook as evenly as possible.

Grill each side, of each of the chicken breasts for approximately 15 minutes, or until chicken is cooked all the way through. There should not be any pink in the center of any of the chicken breasts.
4 ounce serving :   150 calories   5g fat   26g protein

Wasabi Chicken Breast**

Fresh baked or left over chicken breast * (quick and easy!)
Wasabi Sauce
Balsamic Glaze

Here is a way to spruce up the normally boring left over chicken breast you are about to eat for lunch! Wasabi sauce and balsamic glaze do add a small amount of calories, sugars, and fat to the food so only use the finest drizzle. You may want to add a little less than is in the picture, especially less balsamic glaze.
If you want to eat the chicken breast with corn, please make sure it is organic and non-GMO (Genetically Modified Organisms). Most corn is GMO unless it mentions that it isn't on the package, or unless you grew it yourself from heirloom seeds.

Total Calories: 159 calories   2g fat   26g protein   7g carbs

What to do with White Fish**

Another super-lean meat, a staple food for bodybuilders and people looking for fat loss and muscle building results combined. Paired with steamed broccoli, cauliflower, zucchini, or other vegetables and a measured carbohydrate such as brown rice or sweet potatoes, this can be a winning dinner. What is important about these foods are the amounts to be eaten. Please consult a sports nutritionist such as myself for the correct amounts of each food for you.

Pre-heat oven to 400 degrees and coat a baking sheet with non-fat cooking spray.
Take 16 oz. of cod (approximately 4 pieces) and rinse it off in the sink with cold water, then place each piece of cod on baking sheet.

Coat each piece of fish with approximately 1 tsp of extra virgin olive oil. This will allow seasonings to stick to the fish.
Sprinkle the following spices over the surface of each piece of fish: 1/4 tsp of paprika, 1/4 tsp of garlic powder, 1/4 tsp of sea salt, 1/4 tsp of sweet basil, and 1/8 tsp of black pepper.

Place the baking sheet in the oven and bake cod for 12-15 minutes, or until the meat of the cod will flake apart by touching it with a fork. Serve and enjoy!

Calories are counted for 4 ounces of Cod with oil and seasonings.

Total calories: 133 calories   5.5g fat   20g protein

Baked Wild Caught Salmon**

Wild caught Salmon provides essential Omega 3 fats which are necessary for many biological functions, such as contributing to a lower blood pressure, reduction in heart disease, decreases inflammation, and provides many other health advantages. It is important that the salmon is wild, because the farmed salmon is fed a diet that does not contribute to the meat containing the valuable omega 3 fatty acids. Salmon has a sweet, moist red or dark pink flesh that should never taste or smell fishy. Salmon pairs well with sweet potatoes, brown rice, wild rice, or the exotic red Wehani rice (pictured), along with veggies such as broccoli, yellow squash, green beans, spinach, etc. The leftover skin can be ripped up and put in pet food. A tiny 1x1" square piece can go a long way towards a shiny coat and healthy joints for cats and dogs alike.

Pre-heat oven to 400 degrees. Spray a baking sheet with non-fat cooking spray and set pan aside. Take 16 oz. of wild caught salmon and

cut it into 4 evenly sized pieces. Coat the surface of each piece of salmon with 1/2 tsp of extra virgin olive oil.
Sprinkle about 1/2 tsp of Chef Paul Prudhomme's Magic Salmon Seasoning, on top of each piece of salmon.
Sprinkle 1/4 tsp of ground cumin over the top of each piece of salmon. Place pieces of salmon of baking sheet and bake in the oven for 15-20 minutes. Remove skin carefully with a sharp metal spatula and serve.
Makes 4 servings.
Calories for one 4 oz. serving of the salmon alone: 256 calories
16g fat   23g protein

Shrimp cocktail * (Pictured)

14 medium boiled shrimp   101 calories   144mg cholesterol   2g fat
19g protein   1g carb
½ cup ketchup (preferably organic) 116 calories   .5g fat   2g protein   30g carb
2-3 tbsps. deli horseradish (not horseradish sauce) to taste. 8 -12 calories   2-3g carb

While shrimp are high in cholesterol and ketchup is very high in sodium, there are worse things you can treat yourself to.
If you are watching your cholesterol or sodium this snack may not be for you, but if you are reasonably healthy and have no cholesterol or high blood pressure then this is something to pick at while at a party.

Bear in mind, you are also not going to be consuming the entire serving of cocktail sauce.
This homemade sauce tastes much better than bottled cocktail sauce and is a Long Island recipe, which has a large seafood eating culture.
Just boil and peel the shrimp (or buy pre boiled and peeled), pour the ketchup into a small bowl and mix in horseradish slowly, adding more as needed (to taste).

Chapter 4: Entrees

Tacos **

1 Lb. ground or cubed chicken, ground turkey, or lean ground beef
1 cup chopped Lettuce
1 can diced tomatoes with chilies
½ pack of reduced fat Mexican cheese
1 avocado
½ onion, diced
1-2 tbsps. Taco seasoning
1 tbsp. chili powder
Black olives and jalapenos if desired
Low carb whole wheat wraps (we are using nutritional info for Mission Carb Balance wraps here)

Brown ground meat in a skillet sprayed with nonstick spray and mix with taco seasoning, chili powder, and onion. Simmer on medium-low for 3-5 minutes; add a teaspoon of water if mixture is too dry. When cooking is done, drain water. You will most likely have left overs for a taco salad tomorrow. Warm the tortilla in an oven or toaster oven for a few short minutes, then add finely chopped lettuce and spread onto wrap. Add cheese, meat, and tomatoes; be sure to only fill the tortilla a quarter of the way so you will be able to fold it (if that matters to you).

Fold the tortilla in at the side ends until they almost touch, use your thumbs to bring up the bottom of the tortilla tightly. From here on you will roll the tortilla from the bottom up while pulling towards you as you go. Lightly squeeze and bend it and it should stay rolled.

 For a leaner taco, use ground turkey breast rather than plain ground turkey and less or no cheese.

Makes 5 Servings
Total per taco (Filling only)   291 calories   17g fat   35g protein
7g carb   2g fiber
Low Carb Wrap   60 Calories   2g Fat   5g protein
12g carb   7g fiber
Total Nutrition per serving: 351calories   19g fat   35g protein
19g carb   9g fiber

Turkey Muffins **

This recipe was inspired by a recipe by Mandi Grantham and the Facebook group Moms with Muscles.

1 pack ground turkey 20 oz./1.25 lb.
1 cup cooked brown rice
1 whole egg
4 egg whites
2 Tbsp. parmesan cheese
½ medium onion
½ green pepper
¼-1/2 tsp Garlic, 1/8-1/4 tsp black pepper, ¼ cup chopped fresh basil, ¼ cup spinach, ¼ cup fresh chopped parsley, 1/8th tsp sea salt, other spices as desired.
Mix ingredients in a bowl and put mixture in muffin tin sprayed with non-stick cooking spray, bake 40 min @ 330 degrees
Total Cal for 6 servings: 1300 calories   135.5g protein   49g Fat   56.9g carb
Per Serving: 216 calories   22.5g protein   8.1g Fat   9.5g carb
*to save calories, use 1 slice of Ezekiel bread instead of rice. Instead of 218 calories, using the bread gives you:
Bread nutrition: 80 calories   4g protein   .5g fat   15g carbs   3g fiber
Total w/ Ezekiel Bread: 1160 calories   135g protein   47.5 fat   30g carbs
Per Serving (1 of 6 muffins) 196 calories   22.5g protein   8g fat   5g carbs

*to save on the amount of calories per serving, use ground turkey breast instead of plain ground turkey. Save 7g fat per serving; and about 63 calories.

Southwestern Chicken Cakes **
These are made the same as turkey muffins but taste different.
1 pack of ground chicken (or turkey)   20 oz./1.25 lb.
1 cup cooked brown rice
1 whole egg
4 egg whites
½ medium onion
1 green pepper

1/3 can tomatoes with green chilies
2 tsp Penzey's (or other brand) taco seasoning
1 tsp chili powder
½ tsp cumin

Mix ingredients in a bowl and put mixture in muffin tin sprayed with non-stick cooking spray, bake 40 min @ 330 degrees
If desired, you may garnish with a few slices of avocado or salsa; just factor in the added calories.
Total nutrition for 6 servings 1,162 calories   107.5g protein   47g fat   65.4g carb
Per Serving (1 cake) 194 calories   18g protein   8g fat   11g carb
Avocado – 1 whole (1/3-1/2 as a suggested)   234 calories   3g protein   21.4g fat   12.5g carb   10g fiber
Salsa   ¼ cup   17 calories   1g protein   4g carb

Spanish Rice**

(Pictured on the page with Asian Stir Fry and Italian Chicken and Zucchini)
16 oz. of extra lean ground beef or turkey
2 cups of cooked brown rice
1 cup of diced tomatoes.
2 TBSP of tomato sauce
Medium sized onion.
3 cloves of garlic.

Total nutrition: 1414 calories   142g protein   37g fat   118g carb   10g fiber
Recipe makes 4 servings. Each serving contains:
353 calories   35.5g protein.   9.25g fat   29.5g carb   2.5g fiber

Dice up 1 medium sized onion, along with 3-4 cloves of garlic, and place them in a food storage bag. At this time, you will also begin to prepare cooking brown rice on the stove-top according to directions on package. Cook enough brown rice to equal 2 cups after it is cooked.

Add the following spices to the bag of diced onions and garlic: 2 tsp of chili powder, 1 tbsp. of garlic powder, 1 tsp of paprika, 1 tsp of sea salt, 1/2 tsp of cumin, 1/2 tsp of black pepper, 1/2 tsp of cilantro, and 1/2 tsp of onion powder.

Brown 1 pound of extra lean ground beef, chicken, or turkey in a large frying pan at a medium heat. When meat is almost cooked, drain any residual grease from the frying pan, and return it to the burner on the stove.

Empty bag of diced onion, garlic, and spices into the meat. Using a spatula, shuffle all of the ingredients together until everything is evenly cooked.

Add 1 cup of diced tomatoes to the frying pan with meat, onion, garlic, and spices.

Add 2 TBSP of tomato sauce to the frying pan as well. Mix diced tomatoes and tomato sauce in thoroughly with the rest of the ingredients. Allow to simmer until rice is fully cooked. When rice is finished cooking, add 2 cups of cooked brown rice to the frying pan and thoroughly mix it with the rest of the ingredients.
Remove from stove and serve.

Stuffed Pepper Casserole **

1 pack ground turkey 20 oz. /1.25 lb.
1 cup cooked brown rice
2 peppers
1 24 oz. jar tomato sauce
1 6oz can tomato paste
1 medium onion
1 8oz bag low fat mozzarella cheese
½ tsp Garlic powder, ¼ tsp crushed red pepper, 1 tsp oregano, fresh basil
Total: 12 servings   94oz.   2367 calories
190.5g protein 101.5g fat   165.8g carb
Per 8 oz. /1 cup serving: 197 calories
16g protein   8.5g fat   14g carb

Brown turkey in a pan, cook rice as to directions, then combine turkey, pre-cooked rice, sauce, paste, diced or chopped onion and pepper, and spices in large oven safe bake-ware. Sprinkle cheese over top and bake 30 min @ 350 or until cheese is golden. To add more protein to the meal simply add ½ to 1 more package of ground turkey or chicken to the recipe. *To lessen the fat, use ½ pack of cheese and ground chicken breast. To lower the carb content according to your diet, reduce or eliminate the rice.

This meal is a crowd pleaser and will make the whole family happy! It is great to freeze and take to work as leftovers or have for nights afterwards. We brought it to a holiday party and came home with an empty bowl!

Mom's Italian Meat Sauce. Eat it and weep. ***

Classico or Newman's Own, or Organic Tomato sauce Tomato Basil Flavored 2-24 oz. jars
Tomato paste 18 oz. can
2 packs 20 oz. 1.25lb ground turkey 93%lean
Sweet Italian Turkey Sausage 20 oz. (5 links)
Hot Italian Turkey Sausage 14 oz. (3 Links)
1 red pepper, 1 cup chopped
1 green pepper, 1 cup chopped
1 medium yellow onion, 1 cup chopped
3 pinches of sugar
3 cloves of garlic (or 1/2 tsp powder)
Fresh Basil *8 oz. fresh, 1 tbsp. dried
1Tbsp oregano, ¼ tsp crushed red pepper

Total: 20-1cup servings 161 oz.   4211 calories   433g Protein   180g Fat   219g carb*
Serving: 1 cup/8oz 210.55 calories   22g Protein   9g Fat   11g carb*
Optional: Can be eaten over whole wheat pasta, brown rice, or over chopped pan seared zucchini
Whole Wheat Pasta 1 cup cooked, add: *1 cup   174 calories   7.5g Protein   1g Fat   37g carb*
Brown rice 1 cup cooked, add: *1 cup   218 calories   4.5g Protein   2g Fat   46g carb*
Zucchini 1 cup cooked, add: *1 cup   20 calories   1.5g Protein .2g Fat   4.2g carb*

Take the sausages and squeeze the meat out of the casing into 1" cubes in a large pan, add ground turkey and brown all of the meat lightly until most of the pink goes away. Don't take out the water from this. Add chopped or diced onion and pepper. Cook a few minutes. Add tomato sauce in the jars but NOT the paste. We will save that til later. Press and add garlic, stir. Add 1 tbsp. oregano, 3 pinches of sugar, ¼ tsp crushed red pepper; stir, cover, and simmer for 1 hour. Spoon out any

fat (there won't be very much if using turkey products). Add tomato paste, stir, let simmer for 15-30 more minutes, and you are eating for the next week!
*To lower the sodium, use more ground turkey instead of sausages, or use ½ the amount of sausages.

A recipe from Desirée's mother, this one is a real crowd pleaser. This will go over really well with anybody who likes Italian food. It's even good cold and can be eaten without pasta. A recent development has found this sauce is even better with brown rice mixed in than pasta.

Enchiladas **

Mission Low carb whole wheat tortilla (1)
20 oz./ 1.25lb ground turkey/extra lean ground beef
1 8oz can tomato sauce
½ can diced tomatoes with green chilies
1 8oz pack of low fat Mexican cheese
1 packet Mc Cormick Enchilada seasoning
Total (filling only) 5 8oz. servings   40 oz. 1748 calories   173g Protein   88.5g fat   55g carb
1 8oz/1 cup serving no tortilla   350 calories   34.54g Protein   17.7g fat   11g carb
1 serving w/ tortilla   430 calories   37.54g Protein   19.7g fat   37g carb

You will need: 1 package of low carb tortillas, 1 pound of lean ground chicken, or extra lean ground beef, 1 8 oz. can of tomato sauce, 1.5 cups of water, 1 package of shredded low fat Mexican cheese, 1 packet of Mc Cormick Enchilada seasoning, 1 tsp of ground chili powder, 1/2 can of diced tomatoes with green chili peppers (optional).
Stir Sauce Mix, chili powder, water and tomato sauce in medium saucepan. Bring to boil. Reduce heat and simmer 5 minutes or until thickened, stirring occasionally.
Brown meat in large skillet on medium-high heat. Drain fat. Stir in ½ cup of the sauce.
Skim tortillas with sauce until they are lighted coated on each side.
Spoon about 1/4 cup of meat filling into each tortilla. Add about a table spoon full of diced tomato & green chili combo. Add a sprinkle of cheese. Roll tortillas tightly. Place seam-side down in greased 11x7-inch baking dish. Pour remaining sauce over enchiladas. Sprinkle tops of enchiladas with cheese. Bake in preheated 325 °F oven for about 15 minutes, or until sauce is bubbly and cheese is melted.
*to lessen the fat, use ½ the pack of cheese rather than the whole pack; and use ground chicken breast. *to save sodium, replace enchilada

seasoning with cumin, onion powder, and garlic powder, and cilantro if desired.

Lettuce Enchiladas **

Spray skillet or frying pan with non-fat cooking spray. Begin by browning 1 pound of 95 % lean ground chicken in skillet, or frying pan. While ground chicken is cooking, take a medium sized sauce pan, and add 1 can of tomato sauce, and 1/2 cup of water. Turn on burner to bring to a boil. While sauce is heating up, slowly sprinkle in 1/2 packet of enchilada seasoning mix, and 1 TBSP of ground chili powder. Stir frequently to mix in spices. When sauce reaches a boil, then turn down heat to a simmer.
After sauce is thoroughly mixed, scoop up 3/4 cup of sauce from sauce pan, and then add it to the ground chicken after it is cooked. Stir the sauce in with the ground chicken, and mix thoroughly. Let the ground chicken and sauce mixture simmer.

Take 1 head of iceberg lettuce, and peel apart 6 large lettuce leaves. Leaves may be doubled up, depending on how thick of a lettuce coating you would like to use. Lay the lettuce leaves nice and flat on plates, as though they were actually tortillas. Scoop the ground chicken out of the skillet, or pan, and divide the chicken into approximately 6 servings. Place each serving of ground chicken down the center of a large lettuce leaf, or stacked leaves. Take approximately 36 grams of shredded, low fat, 2% cheese, and divide the cheese into 6 servings. Take each serving of cheese, and sprinkle them on top of each serving of ground chicken, which will be placed on the lettuce. Fold, and roll each serving of lettuce, so that they wrap all the way around the ground chicken, and the cheese that was placed on top of them.
When you're finished, you shouldn't be able to see any of the ground chicken, or cheese, as it will all be wrapped in the lettuce, just like a tortilla. Take the remaining sauce off of the burner, and pour it over the top of each lettuce wrapped enchilada. Try to even out the sauce over the 6 enchiladas. In order to make this recipe more visually appealing, you may add a light sprinkle of shredded cheese on top of the sauce covering each enchilada, but be sure to consider the calories that are in whatever amount of cheese that you decide to use.
Serve and enjoy!

1 pound of ground chicken (95% lean)
1 head of Iceberg lettuce
Enchilada seasoning (1/2 packet)
1 can tomato sauce
Enchilada Seasoning 1/2 packet
1 can of Tomato Sauce
1 TBSP Chili powder

Shredded 2% Low Fat Cheese (36 grams).

Makes 6 Enchiladas. Each serving (1 enchilada) contains approximately:
154 calories   5 g fat   18g protein   7 g carb

Italian Chicken and Zucchini **

1 jar quality organic tomato sauce
1 can diced tomatoes
1 package of Italian seasoned ground chicken
2 cups zucchini
4 cups cooked whole wheat spaghetti (1 cup for each serving)
½ cup fresh basil
½ tsp garlic powder
¼ tsp. crushed red pepper
1 tbsp. oregano

Slice zucchini into rounds, then ½ rounds, then quarter rounds. Spray a nonstick skillet with nonstick spray and fry until toasted looking.

Start heating the water for the pasta, cover, and bring to a rolling boil. In a separate skillet while zucchini is cooking, brown ground chicken until pink is gone.

Add the jar of sauce, can of tomatoes, all spices, and finished zucchini into a large pot and simmer on low, stirring occasionally. Add pasta to boiling water and cook as per directions.

When pasta is finished, so is the chicken and zucchini. Measure out pasta and pour chicken mixture over it and enjoy! !

Makes 4 servings. Per serving: 370 calories   16g fat   31g protein   33g carbs   2g fiber

Asian Chicken Stir Fry ** (Pictured)

1 lb. chicken breast	2 tsps. Sesame oil
3 cups of Broccoli	1 tsp. ground ginger
2 cups cooked sprouted brown rice	2 tsps. Asian fusion seasoning
1 pepper	¼ cup soy sauce
1 medium onion	

Chop chicken into chunks, marinate in a gallon sized Ziploc bag, then seal the bag and shake to coat everything. You can let it sit for a couple of hours if desired.

Set rice up to cook.

Stir fry on medium heat in a large skillet, turning for ½ hour. Once chicken is no longer pink than cook veggies in a separate skillet. Use nonstick cooking spray to prevent things from sticking to the pan.

Makes 4 servings.

Calories in one serving: 441 calories   10.5g fat   31g protein
62.5g carb   3g fiber

Chapter 5: Drinks & Shakes

Weight and fat loss is most effective when you can drink as much water as you possibly can, as it keeps you full. You may feel hungry, when in fact you are actually thirsty. Plus, muscles are made of water, so if you are looking to build muscle, water is absolutely essential. Many nutritionists will suggest you drink a gallon or more per day. It is not only good for fat loss, but good for the skin and many other body processes as well. It washes away toxins, maintains digestive regularity, prevents cramps, and cleans your body tissues. It also boosts your immune system, so you will catch colds less often, if at all. Your body is over 70% water, and not drinking enough can give you a dehydration headache. Drinking a gallon of water is something you will have to build up to over a period of a week or two, so no need to run to your faucet immediately after reading this and try to guzzle like a mad person. Your body needs time to adjust. It is also wise to cut off water shortly after dinner so you aren't up all night. If you are the type of person that gets up during night for a trip to the bathroom, you may find over time that drinking more water overall may actually ease that or even end it altogether.

Tips for consuming more water:

*Herbal teas

*Eating watery vegetables such as celery and cucumbers

*Drink a glass of water before and with each meal

*Add lemon, they now have lemon in packets

*Water filters make water much cheaper if you can't drink from the tap

*Drinking through a straw makes you drink more, and drink faster

Flavored Water *

12-16 oz. water

Sweetener of choice: stevia, monk fruit, and Splenda are no-calorie sweeteners. Please use these judiciously, as they are always finding something wrong with sweeteners. Please do NOT use aspartame (usually in a blue packet).
Flavor ideas, you can find these as baking extracts in the baking aisle: Vanilla, blueberry, pineapple, coconut, peppermint, lemon, raspberry, strawberry, banana, and cherry.

You can mix a couple; vanilla goes well with blueberry, banana, mint, any berry, coconut, or pineapple. I have found the orange, chocolate, and peanut butter to taste somewhat artificial.

With the exception of the mint flavors, most flavors are as measured: ¾-1 capful to 12-16 oz water, start with less and add more as desired. Vanilla can be added as much as 1 tsp, but any of the mints are very strong and you only need a few drops. The mint flavored waters seem to sooth upset stomachs as well.

Zero calories *Truvia brand Stevia adds about 2 calories but yields the best taste in my opinion.

Apple Water*

Take 1 liter of filtered water, slice an apple and put the slices in it with a stick of cinnamon. Let it sit in the refrigerator for a day or day or so for some wonderfully calorie free apple flavored water.

Liquid Pumpkin Pie *

½ can pumpkin; no sugar added
1 scoop of your favorite vanilla whey protein
½ tsp vanilla extract
½ cup water
1/8th tsp ginger, cloves, and allspice
¼ tsp cinnamon
4-6 small ice cubes
Add ½ scoop vanilla casein if desired.
Ingredients make one serving.
Total without casein   203 calories   27.5g
protein   1g fat   21.5g carbs   5g fiber
Total with casein   258 calories   39.5g
protein   2g fat   23.5g carbs   5.5g fiber

Put the ½ cup water in blender first, then add sweetener if desired
(since protein is already sweetened, you may not need it at all.
Otherwise we would use stevia or monk fruit). Then add ice cubes,
vanilla, dry spices, protein, then pumpkin.
Blend well making sure Ice cubes are chopped down as much as
possible. If adding casein, bear in mind that will thicken shake up, so if
you like a more watery shake then add ¼ cup more water. You can also
add water incrementally as desired after mixture is blended. If you
prefer a thick, creamy shake then don't add any water on top of the ½
cup mentioned in the ingredient list. This is more than a drink; it is
complete and can be a meal replacement.

Skinny Hot chocolate *
1 tbsp. unsweetened cocoa powder 1 tsp vanilla
6 oz. water
2 oz. unsweetened plain or vanilla almond milk
Sweetener of choice
Add cocoa powder, sweetener, and vanilla to a mug. Boil water, pour
into mug stirring well. Add almond milk.
Yields: 32 calories   2g fat   3g carb   1g protein

Chapter 6: Pizzas

Low Carb Pizza *

Place 1 low carb tortilla onto a baking sheet, and apply 1/4 cup of pizza sauce to the tortilla. Spread evenly over the tortilla's surface. Sprinkle 1/4 cup of low fat 2% shredded cheese evenly over the sauce. Take 1/2 of a sweet Italian turkey sausage link, ripped into small chunks, and place the chunks of meat on top of the shredded cheese.

Take 1/2 of green pepper diced into pieces, and sprinkle the pieces over the top of the pizza. Cut 3 medium sized mushrooms into slices and place them on top of the pizza. Take about 1/2 cup of fresh chopped spinach and sprinkle it on top of the pizza.

Place baking sheet into oven that has been pre-heated to 400 degrees. Bake for 10-15 minutes. Serve and enjoy!

1 serving = 1 pizza: 269 calories   12 grams fat
18g carb   21g protein   9 g fiber

Quick and Easy Mexican Pizza **

1 Angelic Bakehouse Flazza brand flat bread	1 small can green chilies
¾ of a 20 oz. package of ground turkey or chicken	1 Tbsp. Taco seasoning
2 tsps. Chili powder	½ cup pizza sauce
¼ large onion diced, or ½ medium onion	½ cup Diced pre-cooked zucchini
½ 8 oz. package (4 oz.) of Low fat Mexican cheese	1 can of diced tomatoes with green chilies

Brown ground chicken in a pan over medium heat and add taco seasoning and chili powder. Preheat oven to 400 degrees. Spray a pizza pan with nonstick spray and put Flattza bread on it. Spread pizza sauce on Flatzza, sprinkle cheese evenly, and then put the ground chicken on top. Evenly add the onion, diced tomatoes, chilies, and zucchini and cook at 400 for 10 minutes. Makes4 servings; 1 serving is ¼ of the pizza.

Nutrition per serving: 372 calories   16.5g fat   34g protein
25g carbs   5g fiber

Pizza from Scratch ***

Lower fat, whole grain pizza crust

2.5 cups of whole wheat flour
1/4 cup of ground flax meal
1 Tbsp. of active dry yeast
1 Tbsp. of olive oil
1/4 Tsp of salt
1 cup of warm water
1 tsp of pizza spice or garlic powder works well too.
½ cup pizza sauce
2 packs low fat mozzarella or Mexican cheese
Total: 2734 calories
150.5g protein   108.3g fat   276.5g carb
Servings 8   342 calories
19g protein   13.5g fat   34.5g carb
Toppings of choice: chopped spinach, mushrooms, and/ or Italian seasoned ground turkey

First: add yeast and oil to 1 cup of warm water and mix together, and then pour into a large bowl. Add 2 cups of whole wheat flour, 1/4 cup of ground flax meal, 1/4 Tsp of salt, and 1 Tsp of seasoning or garlic powder to the bowl and mix all the ingredients together to form dough.

Dough will be slightly wet and sticky. Add the remaining half cup of flour to the dough and knead the dough with your hands until the dough is well mixed and relatively dry.

Place dough on a large greased pizza pan, or divide it among 2 smaller greased pizza pans, then press and flatten the dough out in the pan, or pans, until the you form the desired thickness of the pizza crust that you want.

Next, add the pizza sauce, low fat cheese, and toppings that you like and bake pizza at 400 degrees for approximately 25-30 minutes.

I personally like to use low-fat Mexican cheese, with chopped spinach, mushrooms and Italian seasoned ground turkey. For a crispier crust, bake on a pizza stone.

Low carb, gluten free pizza crust:

4 eggs
1/4 cup of coconut flour
1/4 cup of ground flax meal
1/4 cup of plain Greek yogurt
1 tsp onion powder
1 tsp of oregano
1 tsp of basil
1/3 cup of shredded Parmesan
2 tsp of garlic powder
1/4 tsp of sea salt
½ cup pizza sauce
2 8oz packs of mozzarella cheese
Total 8 servings: *1895 calories
166.69g protein   111.3g fat   55g carb*
Per Serving: 1 slice   *237 calories
21g protein   14g fat   7g carb*

First: whip eggs, yogurt & sea salt together in a bowl. Add coconut flour and flax meal, and then whip until smooth. Blend in onion powder, oregano, basil, garlic powder and Parmesan. Pour batter onto large greased pizza pan and flatten crust to desired thickness.

Bake at 400 degrees for 10 minutes, then remove from oven and add sauce, cheese, and whatever topping you like. I used spinach, low fat mozzarella, Italian turkey sausage, and black olives.

After you apply the toppings, put back into the oven and bake for an additional 8-10 minutes

Chapter 7: Breads and Desserts

Gluten Free Flax Bread **

2 cups flax seed meal
1 Tablespoon baking powder
1 teaspoon salt
1-2 Tablespoons sugar equivalent from artificial sweetener
5 beaten eggs
1/2 cup water
1/3 cup oil (I use grape seed oil).

Preheat oven to 350 F. Prepare pan (a 10X15 pan with sides works best) spray with Pam spray or line with parchment paper.
Mix dry ingredients well -- a whisk works well. Add wet to dry, and combine well. Make sure there aren't obvious strings of egg white hanging out in the batter.

Let batter set for 2 to 3 minutes to thicken up some (leave it too long and it gets past the point where it's easy to spread. Pour batter onto pan. Because it's going to tend to mound in the middle, you'll get a more even thickness if you spread it away from the center somewhat, in roughly a rectangle an inch or two from the sides of the pan (you can go all the way to the edge, but it will be thinner).

Bake for about 20 minutes, until it springs back when you touch the top and/or is visibly browning even more than flax already is.

Cool and cut into whatever size slices you want. You don't need a sharp knife; I usually just cut it with a spatula.
Nutritional Information: Each of 12 servings has less than a gram of effective carbohydrate (.7 grams to be exact) plus 5 grams fiber, 6 g protein, and 185 calories.

12 Servings
Nutrition per serving: 185 Calories
13g fat   7g Protein   1g carb   6g fiber
*To lessen the fat content, use egg whites, or egg whites with one or two yolks.

Gluten Free Pumpkin Bread **

1 cup of almond flour
1 serving of vanilla whey protein

1/4 cup of flax meal
1/2 cup of pumpkin
3 eggs
1/4 cup of sugar free vanilla syrup
1/4 stick of melted butter
1 tsp of vanilla extract
1/4 tsp of sea salt
1/2 tsp of baking soda
2 tbsp. of cinnamon
1 tsp of pumpkin pie spice
1 tsp of all-spice
1 tsp of ginger
1/4 cup of granulated monk fruit or Splenda sweetener

Total Cal   6 4 oz. servings   24oz   1301 calories   68.2g
protein   103.5g fat   63.5g carb   19g fiber
Per Serving: 4 oz. slice   216 calories   11.4g
protein   9.3g fat   10.58g carb   6g fiber

This bread is high in protein, fiber, antioxidants and essential fatty acids. Here is how you make it: Mix dry ingredients. Next: mix wet ingredients in a separate bowl: 1/2 cup of pumpkin, 3 eggs, 1/4 stick of melted butter, 1/4 cup of sugar free vanilla syrup, and 1 tsp of vanilla extract.

Add wet ingredients to dry ingredients and mix. Pour into bread pan and bake at 350 degrees for 30-35 minutes.

Chad's Gluten Free Cheesecake ***

Pie Crust: Mix these dry Ingredients in a bowl:

2 cups almond flour

½ cup ground flax meal

1 tsp cinnamon

1 tbsp. Splenda

½ tsp baking soda

½ tap salt

Next, mix these wet Ingredients:

½ cup low fat butter (land O lakes Light)

1 egg

2 tbsps. Sugar free vanilla syrup

Total calories   2145 calories   195g fat

67g protein   69g carb

Combine and mix wet & dry ingredients well, then place batter in a pie tin and press batter into the pan to form crust. Use a fork to give a design to the edge by pressing tangs into it all the way around crust. Bake at 325 degrees for 15-20 minutes.

Cheese Filling:

64 grams (2 scoops) of whey protein (the best results have some from CSN Pro-Whey brand whey protein in Vanilla or Vanilla Ice Cream flavor.

41 (1 1/3 scoop) grams of Casein (the best results have some from The Vitamin Shoppe's brand Body Tech in French Vanilla Flavor

8 oz. Low fat cream cheese

1 cup plain Greek yogurt

Total calories: 996 calories   38.5g fat   113g Protein

47g carb

Mix ingredients together with a large spoon and add to cooled pie crust. Chill in refrigerator for 1 hour. If desired, top with fresh fruit & sugar free syrup.

Whole pie, total   3141 calories   233.5g fat   180g Protein 116g carb

Serving (1/10th of the pie) 314 calories   23.35g fat   18g Protein   11.6g carb

Pie Filling Alone (4 servings) 996 calories   38.5g fat   113g Protein   47g carb

1 serving   249 calories   9.6g fat   28g Protein 12g carb

*To save calories, eat the filling without the crust.

Gluten Free Pumpkin Cheesecake Enchilada

This dessert contains fewer calories than the previous cheesecake because there is less crust. The cheesecake enchilada is a fun dessert to bring to parties and is sure to be a crowd pleaser, especially to the gluten free crowd. It is diabetes friendly as well.

Crust crumbles:
½ cup almond meal
¼ cup ground flaxseed
¼ tsp. salt
2 tbsp. Monk fruit powder
1 tsp cinnamon
¼ tsp. baking soda
2 tbsp. sugar free syrup (we use Smucker's or Walden Farms)
1 tsp. vanilla extract
1 egg
1/8 cup melted Smart Balance Spread

Cheesecake filling:
8 oz. low fat cream cheese
2 scoops vanilla whey protein
1 scoop vanilla casein
1/3 cup canned pumpkin
1 cup plain nonfat Greek yogurt
1 tsp. cinnamon
½ tsp. allspice
¼ tsp. cloves
¼ tsp. nutmeg

Pre-heat oven to 325 degrees. In a large bowl combine the following dry ingredients: Almond meal flour, ground flax seed, Monk fruit powder, cinnamon, salt, and baking soda. Stir together thoroughly. In a small separate bowl, combine the following wet ingredients: Egg, sugar free syrup, vanilla extract, and softened Smart Balance. Beat ingredients together with a fork until all the ingredients are thoroughly blended. Add wet ingredients to bowl of dry ingredients and mix together thoroughly to form batter.

Spray a cookie sheet with non-fat cooking spray. Remove the batter from the bowl and place it on the cookie sheet. It will be moist and sticky. Press down on batter and flatten it out on the cookie sheet. The shape is not important. Just make sure that the batter is pressed down until it resembles a large flat cookie in the cookie sheet. Place cookie sheet in oven and bake for 15-20 minutes, or until the crust on the cookie sheet begins to brown.

While crust is baking in the oven, take a large bowl and add the following ingredients to it. 8 oz. of low fat cream cheese, 2 scoops of vanilla whey protein, 1 scoop of vanilla casein protein, 1/3 cup of canned pumpkin, 1 cup of plain, fat-free Greek yogurt, cinnamon, all spice, cloves, and nut meg. If the brand of protein powder that you're using isn't as sweet as you would like, you may add stevia, or monk fruit powder to these ingredients to give the cheese cake filling a sweeter taste. Using a sturdy spoon, mix all of these ingredients together. This will take a few minutes as these ingredients are more solid. Stir until all ingredients are thoroughly mixed. It should have a thick frosting like consistency. Cover bowl with plastic wrap and place in the freezer for approximately 1 hour.

When the crust has finished baking in the oven, remove it from the oven and allow to sit and cool until crust begins to harden. This usually takes 20-30 minutes. After the crust has cooled off and is firm, remove it from the cookie sheet and crumble the entire crust up into crumbs, then place the crumbs in a small bowl and set aside.

After the pumpkin cheese cake filling has been in the freezer for about 1 hour, remove it from the freezer. Pour the bowl of crust crumbs onto cookie sheet that you used to bake the crust. Spread the crumbs out evenly on the cookie sheet.

Using your hands, scoop the cold pumpkin cheesecake filling out of the bowl and form the cheese cake filling into a tubular shape, approximately 7-8 inches long. It should be shaped like a 1 pound sausage. The cheese cake filling will be thick enough from being in the freezer, that you should be able to form it relatively easy.

Once you form the cheese cake filling into the desired shape, place it on top of the crumbs on the cookie sheet and roll it back and forth like a rolling pin, until the entire tube of cheese cake filling is coated in the crumbs, which will serve as a light crust for the pumpkin cheese cake.

The pumpkin cheese cake is now ready to be served. If you plan on serving the cheese cake later on, then place it in the freezer in a freezer safe container. Then remove it from freezer and allow it to thaw out about 1 hour before serving.

Total Nutrition for 8 servings: 1640 calories   95g fat   134g protein   69g carbs   16g fiber
Total Nutrition per serving: 205 calories   11g fat   17g protein   8g carbs   2g fiber

Notes

www.ingramcontent.com/pod-product-compliance
Lightning Source LLC
Chambersburg PA
CBHW050351290526

45785CB00006B/2723